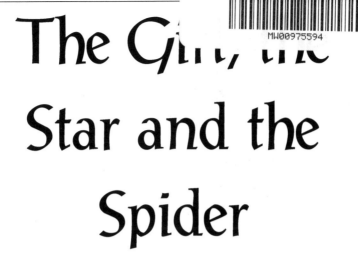

The Girl, the
Star and the
Spider

ىھ A Fairy Tale
for Grownups Dealing with
Alzheimer's and Similar Dementias ﻋﺞ

By Sherry Van Atta Smelley

Illustrated by
Christine Anderson Guldi

The Girl, the Star and the Spider

A Fairy Tale for Grownups Dealing with Alzheimer's and Similar Dementias

Third edition published January 2011

ISBN: 1451504284

EAN-13: 9781451504286

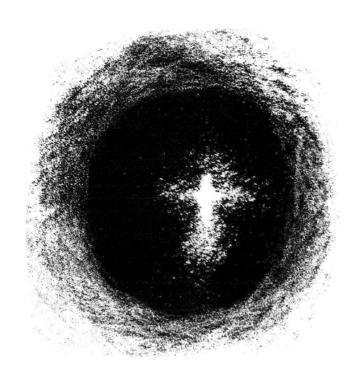

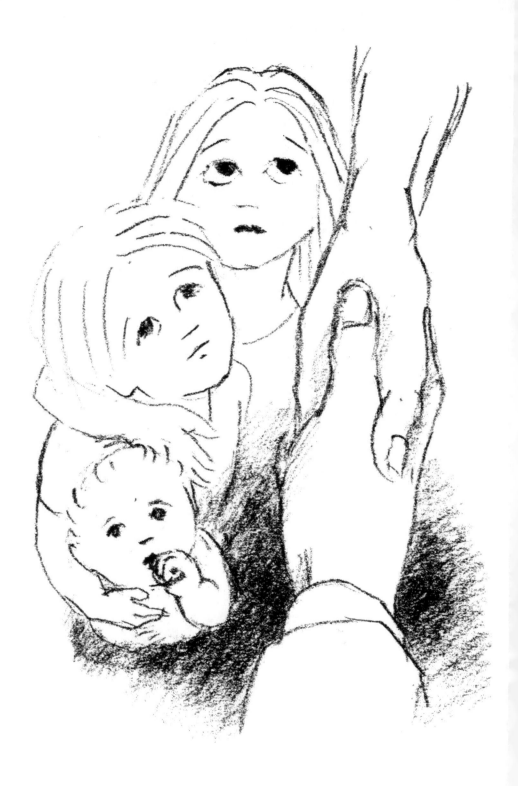

The Girl, the Star and the Spider

Once upon a time . . . a girl was born into a world of darkness and despair. Before she was even ten years old her mother died leaving a dozen children with their poor, poor father who was unable to feed his hungry children. He sent word out to the village that children were "for sale".

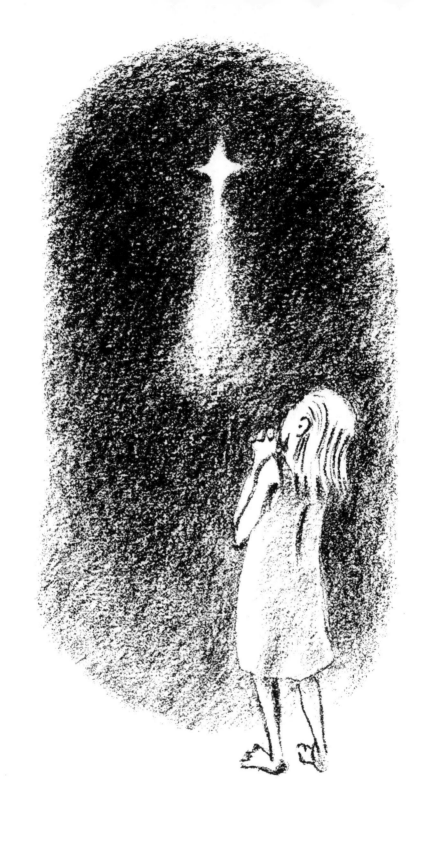

That evening the girl – so afraid of her fate – looked up into the heavens and spotted a star in the night sky, a star brighter than all the rest. She clasped her hands together, closed her eyes and

wished . . .

wished . . .

wished . . .

upon that star. "Please help me, star.

"Please keep me safe.

"Please keep me surrounded by a big love such as my mother's.

"And finally, star, let me one day have my own family and be blessed to live to be old and see all my children grown."

The room grew bright. The girl sensed something present but was almost too afraid to peek.

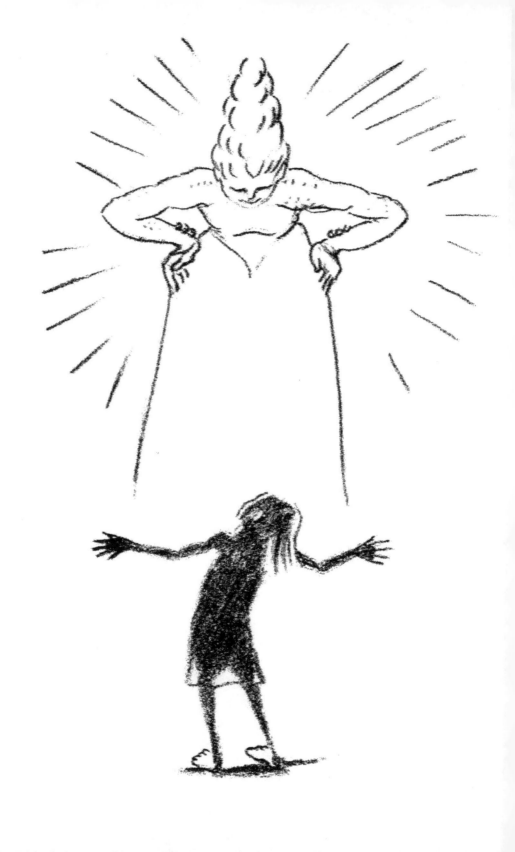

She slowly opened her eyes and there before her was the star. The very star she had just wished upon. The star said, "I heard your plea and have come. I have the power to grant your three wishes but there will be a price to pay." "Anything," the girl said "No price would be too great to be safe, to be surrounded by love this big, and to grow old with my very own family and my children."

"Not so fast" the star said. "You have not heard the price for these."

"Please tell me", she said, "Please tell me."

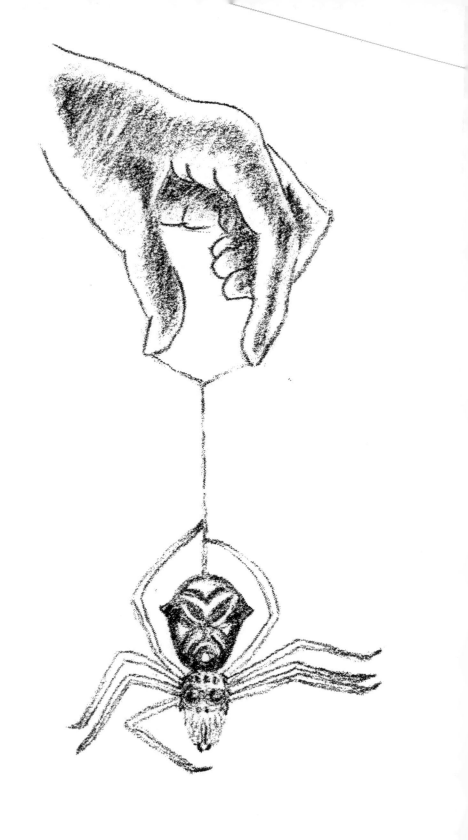

"Oh, you will be safe, you will grow old with your family, and you will have this great love all of your life for others, and they for you . . . but one day when you are old – very, very old – the star spider will come and spin webs in your head . . .

"slowly,

"slowly,

"slowly

stealing your memories." The star nodded as she continued with a serious look on her face.

"You will be safe.

"You will have your family.

"You will love and be loved – a big, big love.

"But by the time you grow very old and die you will remember all this no more."

"I'll take the deal," the girl said. "Sign here" said the star and then rolled up the scroll and disappeared into the night sky.

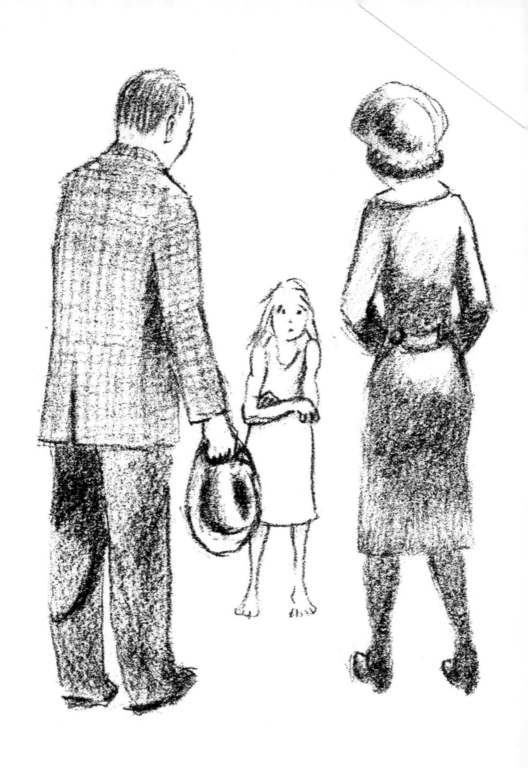

The next day, as
the girl feared, a
strange man and
woman came to
her father's home
and she was
taken away.
They were not
unkind to her.
She had food to
eat, books to
read,

and she grew

and she grew

and she grew.

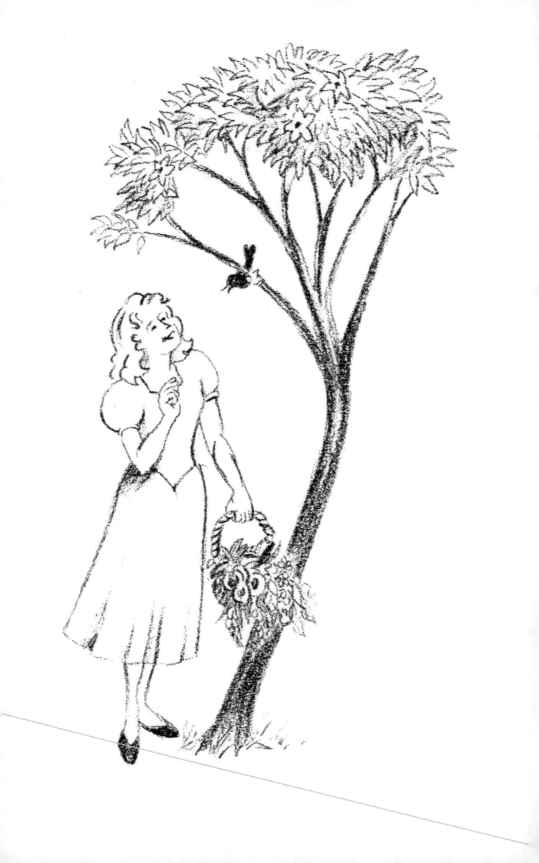

Soon the girl was a young woman and realized that the first wish upon the star had been, in fact, granted . . . so far.

She had been safe.

She then began to consider the second wish and suddenly, almost like magic a handsome young prince appeared. They fell deeply in love and vowed "til death do us part". Children were born, birds sang in her sky and flowers bloomed on her path. She was happy, safe and loved. The gift of the second wish was unfolding.

The girl loved her world and her family and they all loved her.

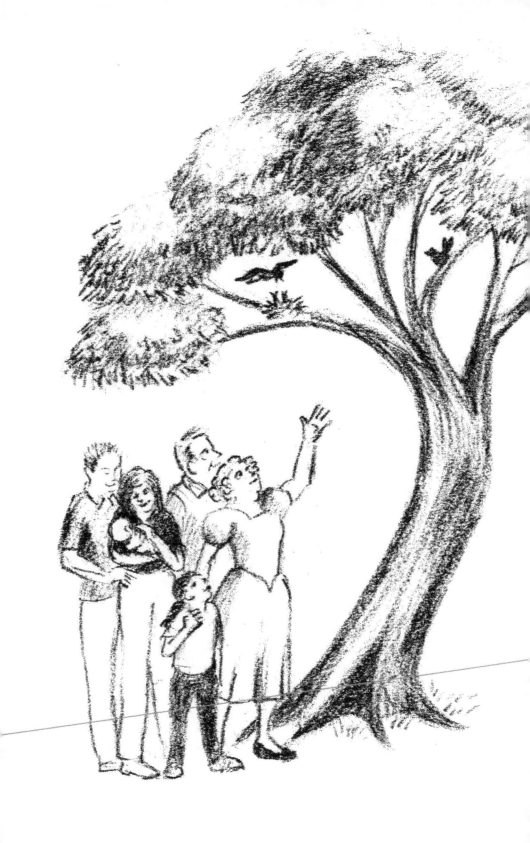

The children grew

and they grew

and even married

and had children of their own.

They often remarked to each other that they felt

so safe and so loved

just being close to their mother, the girl.

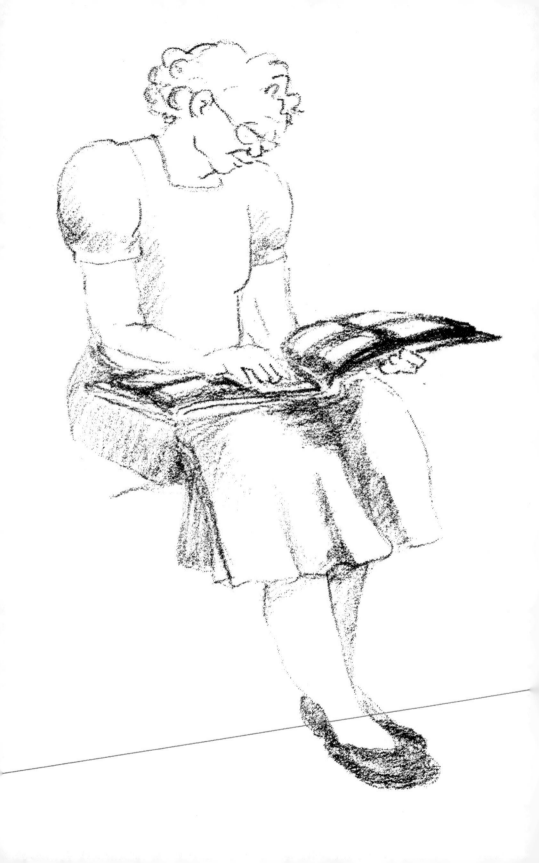

The girl kept the star's visit and her agreement locked carefully in her heart all these years. She told no one, not even the prince. As she grew older, weaker, frailer, she secretly hoped that the star would forget the promise she had made. But no, it was not to be.

> One lovely spring day the girl – now an old woman – heard a knock at the door. There stood the star with the spider at her side. "Please, no" she said, "I do not ever want to forget my family or to leave them. Please do not take my memories." But the star said, "You made a promise and now it is time." The girl understood. She understood a promise – honor, character, courage – these were strong within her. So she said,
>
> "Let it begin."

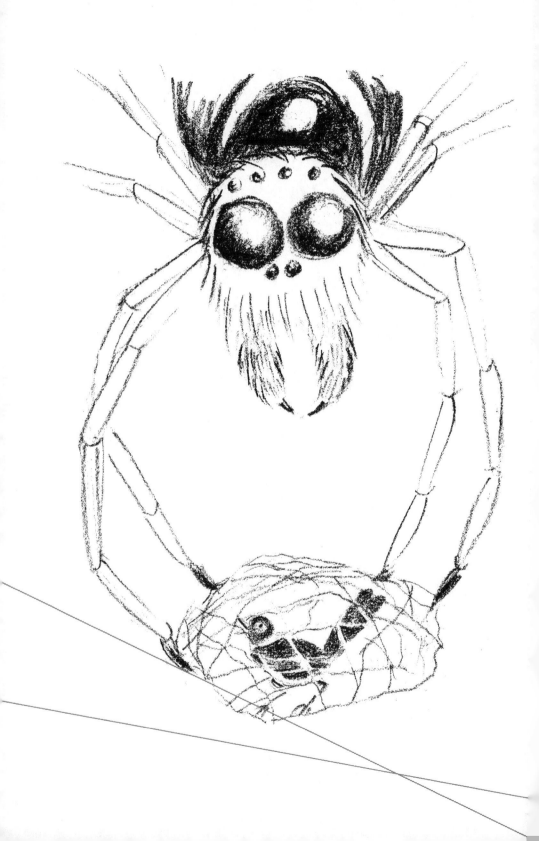

Slowly

ever

so

slowly

the spider began to weave the web
and wall off her memories.

First she could not remember what
she had for lunch, then the way to
the store or if she paid her bills or
washed her clothes.

Yet all of this was okay
with the girl because
she still knew her
family and cherished
their memories.

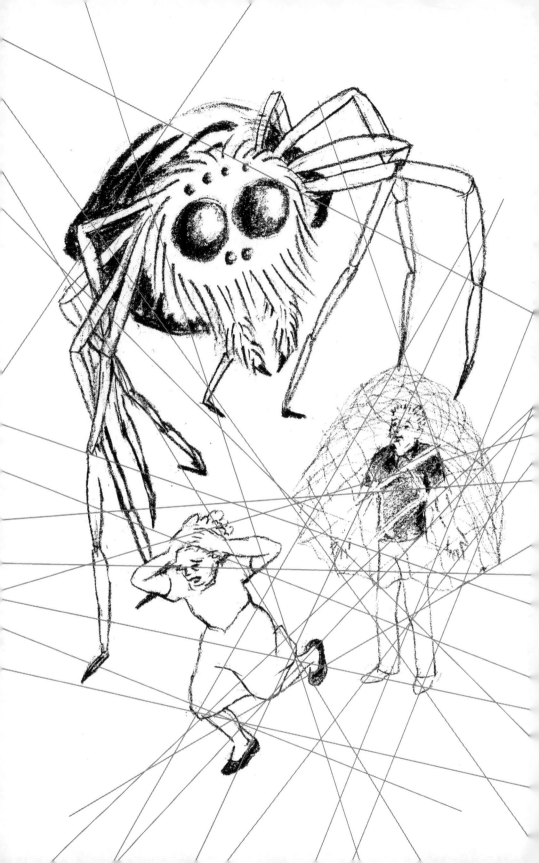

Yet, slowly, slowly even these began to fade.

One dark day her prince left her side and the spider's weaving got faster and faster and her world became dimmer and dimmer . . .

darker and darker.

Her family was so sad and grieved so deeply . . .

day after day, week after week, month after month, year after year the weaving continued.

Finally the day came when she remembered no more . . .

and the star came to take the girl.

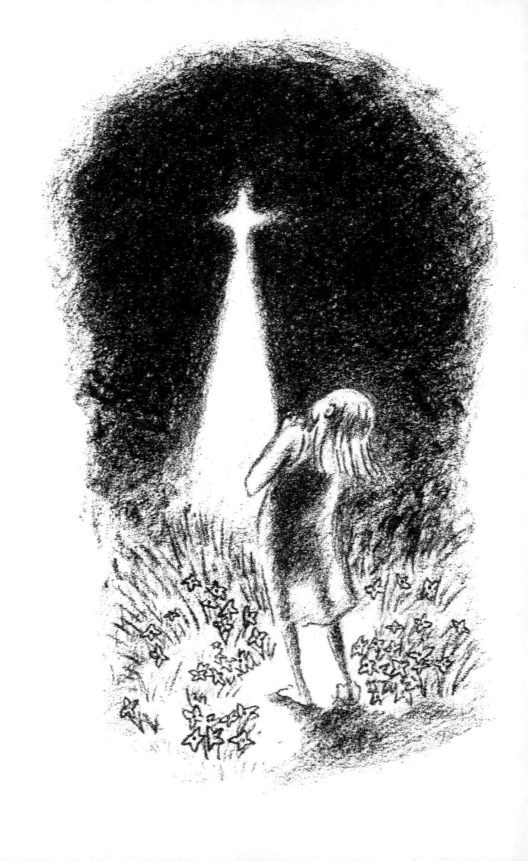

The girl recognized the star immediately!

"I knew how hard this would be for your family and for you," the star said, "Yet a love such as yours could only leave this world a thread at a time. If love the size of yours had left all at once there would have been such a hole that Heaven and Earth would have been sucked in. I knew this when you called upon me all those years ago and realized that to grant your wishes, this would be the only way for you to let go of your family and they of you."

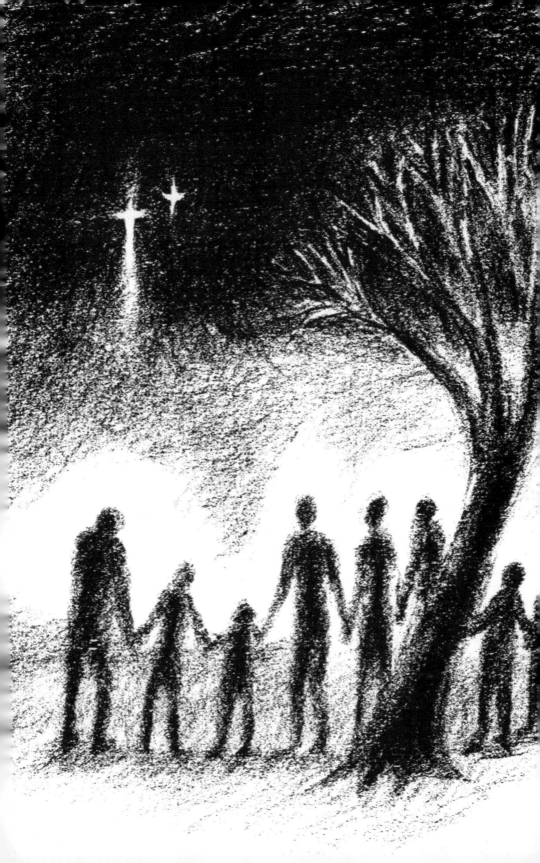

"Look down, girl.

"See, they stand in a circle.

"The brilliant glow around them is the love you left in their hearts. Your love was so strong, so big, it stayed even after you left."

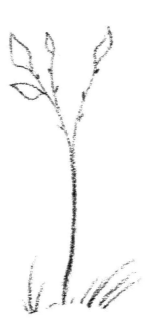

And her family lived happily ever after ... most days. ✍

Afterword

Deeper meaning resides in the fairy tales told to me in my childhood than in any truth that is taught in life. —Friederich Schiller (1759-1805)

As a counselor I work with many adults experiencing grief and loss. In my practice I have utilized numerous methods to help people with their journeys of pain. A few of these are journaling, letter writing, art, poetry, music, and even children's stories. Yes, I read children's stories to adults. I call them "cleverly disguised pieces of adult literature." Part of why I think this medium works is because persons in significant pain are unable to concentrate for very long. Additionally the simplest concepts are the ones that often comfort most. And finally, it could be that the very idea of a children's story takes us back to a place familiar, a place of safety when things were not so dark. Maybe it is a little like going back into our childhoods – re-entering a time when we were tucked safely in our beds and closed our eyes and went to sleep. I know this is how it is for me, remembering a time when my mother read stories – stories of both magic and monsters. So, I read these "children's" stories to clients.

I also teach Grief and Bereavement at the university and have students write children's books on grief as part of the curriculum. At the end of the semester these books are donated to local agencies to be used by the clients. These books become very powerful tools both for the writers and the readers.

Life is full of monsters and magic. My earliest memories of the magic: my mother and books. She read poetry and great pieces of literature to me when I was an infant. By the time I was four years old, I was reading. How I loved it. My mother often took me to the library and I would bring home my own treasures – my favorites were the Fairy Tales. I found delight and comfort in these stories of lost children, witches, dragons, mermaids . . . always beginning with "once upon a time" and ending with "and they lived happily ever after." These stories help us feel comfort by acting as a light in our darkness, giving the illusion of understanding.

A number of years ago my mother began a journey into "the forgetting." She was diagnosed with Alzheimer's disease. The Magic ended. The Monster was unleashed. Grief is the price – the ransom – we pay for love. If we love, we will grieve when that love is lost. Alzheimer's disease and other forms of dementia are different in that the individual disappears slowly, slowly one thread at a time. One memory slips away then another and another and another . . . it is, as we have been told, "the Long Goodbye".

After many years, many tears, my mother died. The emptiness was indescribably painful as was the journey through the disease, a disease so devastating it threatens to rob those left behind of even their good memories. As I sat with my tears and my torment, a story emerged from this darkness. Once again I found that safe place in a fairy tale. "The Girl, the Star and the Spider" was born of my pain. It comforted me. I pray it comforts you.

The Girl, the Star and the Spider may be purchased
online at
www.sherrysmelley.com

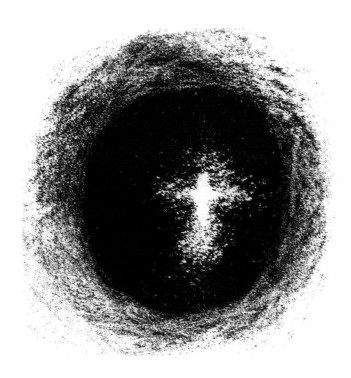

AD is a disease that affects over
five million persons in the US and
is expected to grow to as many at 16
million by 2050. One person is
diagnosed every 71 seconds. By
mid-century, one will be diagnosed
every 33 seconds. The numbers are
staggering. God help us.

Questions for Reflection or Discussion

Alzheimer's Disease Process

1. For many, Alzheimer's Disease can be confusing, often frustrating, and difficult to understand. List questions you have about what happens with this disease.

2. The disease does not progress uniformly but may leave some moments or areas in life apparently disease-free. What has this created for you and what has your response been?

3. How does the gradual onset and slow subsequent decline affect your ability to accept or adjust to its effects in your life or your loved one's life, both in positive and negative ways?

4. How does losing short term memories differ from losing long-term or deep, treasured memories?

5. The spider is scary. Have you experienced fear concerning the disease? How intense is your fear? What aspects of the disease are the scariest to you?

Longevity

1. With today's longer life spans we are often challenged to live with a number of chronic illnesses; we average three by the age of 65. How do we prepare ourselves? Our loved ones? What costs accompany longevity? What opportunities?

2. The girl in the story had a difficult childhood and old age but an apparently charmed adulthood.

What has been the path in your loved one's life? In your own life? What joys, struggles or pain did each of you face? What memories do you treasure most? Is it possible to celebrate both the pains and the joys?

3. The girl was evidently much loved. How is our love for others and theirs for us affected, both positively and negatively, when memories of love disappear?

4. In the end, the old woman is once more pictured as a young girl. Does this correlate with the role reversal of a child caring for an ill parent? Other than the need for care, how might one be a child at any age?

Meanings

1. In the story, the spider's web is the price for having had a long and good life. What meaning would you assign to the disease? Is it a cost of prior blessings, a punishment, a random event? How does the meaning you assign the disease affect your feelings about it?

2. One thread, then a tangle of threads across the page represent the progress of the disease. What images would you use to describe the disease?

3. Does the girl cross gender and cultural lines? How is this story about Alzheimer's Disease like your own story? How might your experience be of value to others?

4. The girl asked a star for help when she was troubled. Where do you turn for help or hope? Do you see hope in this story?

Resources

Alzheimer's Association
225 North Michigan, 17th Floor
Chicago, IL 60601
(312) 335-8700
24/7 Helpline: 1-800-272-3900
www.alz.org

Alzheimer's Disease Education and Referral Center (ADEAR)
P.O. Box 8250
Silver Spring, MD 20907-8250
(301) 495-3311
1-800-438-4380
www.nia.nih.gov/alzheimers

Alzheimer's Disease International
64 Great Suffolk Street
London
SE1 0BL
UK
Tel: +44 20 79810880
www.alz.co.uk

American Health Assistance Foundation (AHAF)
22512 Gateway Center Drive
Clarksburg, MD 20871
1-800-437-2423
www.ahaf.org

AARP
601 E St., NW
Washington, DC 20049
1-888-687-2277
www.aarp.org

American Geriatrics Society
The Empire State Building
350 Fifth Ave., Suite 801
New York, NY 10118
(212) 308-1414
www.americangeriatrics.org

The Cognitive Neurology and Alzheimer's Disease Center
320 East Superior St.
Searle 11-453
Chicago, IL 60611-3008
(312) 908-9339
www.brain.northwestern.edu

National Council on Aging
1901 L Street, NW, 4th floor
Washington, DC 20036
(202) 479-1200
www.ncoa.org

National Family Caregivers Association
10400 Connecticut Ave., #500
Kensington, MD 20895-3944
1-800-896-3650
www.thefamilycaregiver.org

National Institute on Aging
Building 31, Room 5C27
31 Center Drive, MSC 2292
Bethesda, MD 20892
(301) 496-1752
www.nia.nih.gov

U.S. Department of Health and Human Services
Administration on Aging
One Massachusetts Avenue NW
Washington, DC 20201
(202) 619-0724
Eldercare Locator: 1-800-677-1116
www.aoa.gov

National Institute of Neurological Disorders and Stroke
P.O. Box 5801
Bethesda, MD 20824
1-800-352-9424
www.ninds.nih.gov

Made in the USA
Columbia, SC
07 October 2024

43229143R00020